STABILIZER

STABILIZER

Steven Joseph McCrystal

ISBN: 9798851038631

First edition published by Inherit The Earth Publications
©2022
In conjunction with Amazon.

Editor
CT Meek

Steven's latest book deals with his continuous journey from relapse onward. It's a powerful and emotive account of his life to date. Steven's struggle is constant and it's none more so highlighted in his poem The Grudge. It's apparently clear that he considers his past a detoured and warped link to his future and his future a distorted and adulterated pathway back to his past. Steven echoes what many of us feel, what lots of us have experienced, and what a great deal of us are still living through. I believe Steven's core message is that life has to be enjoyed but not taken lightly.

Meek
2022.

Dedicated to any bipolar traveller, or any person who suffers from mental health challenges.

Steven
July
2022

Content -

A Tornado's Kiss

Buckle up

Batten down the hatches

A life force awakens for the uninitiated

From the crack of lightnings

Striking the ground

To the eye of the storm

To the vortex

To the chaos of cows spinning around

Kansas is going bye-bye

Give me shelter

Give me hope

Give me the courage to chase the storm and embrace the joke

It is after all a magic carpet ride into the West

Mother Nature's wrath at its best

A beautiful destruction of heart and home

A chance to rebuild what was lost in the clouds

But who are you after the tempest has gone?

Alien Inside

Do people know?

Do people see it growing inside?

Implanted eggs becoming more than thought

Festering until they are aired

Secrets on the table instead of in your head

Gnawing, changing, choking, morphing, adapting

Staying inside and turning the key

Soul seeking freedom from within

Soul seeking liberation, not a simple whim

A loud voice seeking to break the locks of denial and shame

Open discourse being the ultimate test of self-control

Composure's soul keeps on trying to keep its cool

Who will I be today; I still have a shell to lose?

One of many I've shed as another level up ticks on by

Smile, smile, smile, they won't know what you mean

Public inspection

Anxiety blues

Morbid embarrassment

Diversions and good day platitudes

I will survive this conversation

Maybe I'll wait for my revelations

Freedom of speech without stipulations

But speak to me too because I might be hiding behind the truth

Even if it is a tad uncool and a tad uncouth

Always Look On The Bright Side Of Life

Look at the breath-taking view

Spread-eagled and a little askew

Nails in my hands, I don't give a damn

Sing me a song of salvation if you can

Jesus Christ superstar, I'm not a fan

A fanfare for the common man

Discover the bright side of doom

Bathe in the storms of insanity that brew

Wash the blood from my guts, feet, and hands

Forget the wars if you can

Forget the people killed in his name

He's still our love, he's still our man

Our hearts lifted on the wings of a dove

Always look on the bright side of love

Always look on the bright side of life

I will survive this bloody old strife

Just get drunk my blood is like wine

Eat bread, things will be fine

Because there are so many fishes to find

Cast a net in my infinity pool

Don't use hooks, forget to be cruel

History bought into his deluded dreams

It's a lie, a lie, I want to scream

Forty days without food it seams

A joke, one that's been misunderstood

There lies the insanity and all of the good

Baptiste's instructions for religious clarity

Starve until you hallucinate

Seek the Holy Spirit in your wake

Madness for some, a chemical imbalance

Magic for others with no knowledge of illness

Science facts for this messiah's rites of passage

A mind lost somewhere in the wilderness

Forty days without food it seems

A journey through a desert's delirium

If only he knew simple schoolyard biology

Or even sat in a class of common psychiatry

To clarify the cosmic conundrum of this day

Was Jesus anointed by God, psychosis, thorns, or clarity?

He met the devil it's said, we know that's not true

What other wonders have led us askew?

The magic of miracles I bet, there's been a few

Any Old Rags

One step away from twilight

Two steps away from silence

Past woes and future goals

Timeless connections

I am eternity in recession

The years travel fast

Joy, pleasure, love, pain

Emotions amassed

They are linked to enlightenment

Philosophical hues

A refinement

Just take a sip

Wet your lips

From the chalice of excitement

Drink up your life

Have dreams

Be everything

Scream to go faster

Be the definition of a satisfied disaster

Body Of Lies

Halleluiah, here I am

I'll be your friend

I don't give a damn

Inspiration found on tap

Slap, slap, slap

Growing pains that come with change

When a dull acceptance pounds your brains

Here I am ready for the cull

Denial not an option

Be free, cavort, forget the lies

Seek liberation in honestly

Don't die

Don't be just one more body tossed on the funeral pyre

Don't be a million misplaced words looking for the fire

Be one word in a million

The truth

Be that vital spark

Ignite the lies and embrace the dark

Boogie Nights

Listen to the rhythm feel the beat

Get on the dancefloor move your feet

Lights flashing, music loud

You are dancing in the crowd

People watching all your moves

Fitting right into the grooves

Tunes are playing all night long

Different moves for each song

Dj's cutting on the decks

Up the tempo, feel the sweats

Heart is beating hard and fast

Wonder how long you'll last

Keep it going all night long

On the dancefloor where you belong

When the music's over, turn out the lights

That's it finished for tonight

Conflict

I seek an attitude adjustment

My anger sees only pain

A soul destruction within,

Within these poisons for my mind

I've used the tools of life:

Happiness, joy, reflection, and disdain

I seek an attitude adjustment

Some say Soma for the brain

A prism of light projected,

From a heart that that always craves

A rainbow coloured light

From the darkness that prevails

Does Sex Still Sell?

Hips, tits, and beautiful bums

Buy this car

Buy this fun

Watch this space for perfume ads

Grooming kits for pleats and curls

All or nothing as beauty unfurls

But boys will be boys

Good or bad

Male libidos a selling point

Not a fad

Sex, longing, desire, pleasure

Lovelace on video

Lovelace on cue

Lovelace in view

Men forget

Forget feminism

Forget intelligence

Forget achievement

Forget substance

History tells us to worship beauty

I myself have whistled wolfishly

But somethings have been forgotten

The goddess

The woman

The companion of course

Our mothers were once young and beautiful

Our sisters embraced an unbridled dance

Mother Nature's only chance

To sell sex quietly without a man

Would that ever happen?

Could that ever happen?

It's not been part of the male plan

Since man worshipped sex instead of just being a fan

Drug Of The Nation

Who is glued to the set?

Half the world I would bet

Fantasy worlds

Superhero boys

Superhero girls

Dystopian futures we tried to miss

Reality creatures from the abyss

Mind jacked into our escapes

Jaws open, mind agape

Surely it can't get worse than this

An advert for fear

An advert for bliss

An advert for docudrama

But just hold on my dear

Just hold on

Let's see a horror movie

Right there on your TV

Shocking us right out of our brains

Hands over eyes, hands in a clasp

Unplug, relax, and have look

Let's have a blast

Get a popcorn fright

Get ready to cook

Get ready to fight

But fiction, fantasy; our own creation

Necessities to escape our final destination

Our harsh realities beckon

But television?

The drug of a nation

An overdose of Soma stimulations

Our minds played out for the next generation

The good,

The bad,

The ugly,

The way of the fist

Anything from our twisted imaginations

It is our creation

But what an education

Remote control

We need to escape so what's our destination?

Early Morning Rises

We awaken from a slumbering sleep

Groggy, sober, and full of dreams

Hemispheres in light and shade

Our morning sun which hopes to stay

On its journey, travelling; in and out of sight

Scottish clouds

Mist

Some rains

A passing phase

Traversing through the rays and glades

Summer's sun and winter's night

Muddle through the day

With soulful satisfactions

Eternally Grateful

I give thanks to those friends who fix your heart

Especially to the ones who don't even know it

Strangers yet to be friends, I hope

Their kindness, their patience, their understanding

It changes, we change, and that's a start

Today is the day you changed me

For that I'm eternally grateful

A heartfelt thanks from the depths of my soul

To one and all who know me

Fanny By Gaslight

Really, you don't have to say

Don't look, just push that away

Nothing too big to gaslight by night

Let's all just put that out of sight

Your problems are small

You've only had an insignificant fall

They, that, what will just go away one day

If enough time passes your opinion will sway

Your wounds will heal

Or so they say

Oblivion doesn't matter

Your heart doesn't matter

Only this dim flame of light will guide you in your pain

Yep, that's the game

Follow me around this maze of shite

Pitfalls, problems, pain, and plight

Avoidance of the void at night

Boom, another victim of fanny by gaslight

Fire Starter

I see fire

I close my eyes

I see fire

In my dreams I see the flames

In my dreams I see the world again

In my dreams I see the flames

Cavorting, twisting, spinning, crackling

Dancing

Sparks ascending in the dark

Floating

Flickering

Embracing their ascension

At their heart a furnace

At their heart the flames

For The Love Of Art

What seed sprouts an artistic heart?

One simple idea like I can do that

A desire to express one's very own soul

A connection to you and to all that you feel

A language without words or definitions that's real

A heart full of hunger pounding away

Could it be fun, a day in the sun, a jovial joke in play?

Could it be an obsession of clarity?

Maybe mischief in its own way

Satisfactions gained from getting deep down and dirty

Don't forget that empty head philosophy

Abstraction, passion, perfection

All the heart you can muster

A new edition to the fervour collection

Heart be still, a simple look, other people's hearts are on the hook

I mean everything is art in its own way

Soulful objects come out to play

Artist's hearts put on display

A priceless commodity imagined this day

But what a world it would be with nothing to see?

So why don't you wonder me with your heart my friend

Art, art, art, I hope it never ends

Fortitude

Is there enough endurance left in the world?

I'm scared to watch the news and blues

Hope through medicine. Have a heart

Fortitude, dig deep, don't come apart

We're stuck in solitude

Is there an end in sight?

Can we see or feel the light?

Muddled, distraught, lost in chaos

Will this virus ever obey us?

Is the tunnel far too dark?

To navigate,

To fight,

To have a heart

Will it lose us in this plight?

We must get by this.

We must fight

The long game running is all we know

Fallen friends. Pain and love. We're at a total loss

I'm scared to watch the news and blues

But hope, well that's a start, we need fix this in our hearts

We will beat this. Don't come apart

Glory Days

Meandering in these hot halcyon days

Playing sticks and stones will break my bones

Up a tree and down the gully

Falling down either way

Rambling like there's no tomorrow

Too hot for trouble

Too hot for thrills

Too hot for that last taboo

Sugar and spice and all things nice

This crush can only be true

But bashfulness beats curiosity

It's all about that clumsy confidence

Friends chosen with freedom in mind

Before responsibility

Before BMX health and safety

Big air, 360's, quarter pipes and kick turn ramps

Tough Tarmac fails

Only fifteen and heading off the rails

I had access, my dad had a pub

My friends seeking adventure through libation

No lack of confidence during this consumption

Gone is the innocence of the new

Upon reflection I feel some sorrow

Because memories fade like there's no tomorrow

Heroes Are EZ

A little bit of chaos my friend

Political satires do define,

But EZ just says twats

They should be fined, imprisoned, put in stocks

Their heads placed upon a chopping block

Revolution in our midst

Follow me, I shake my sticks

Heckled endlessly by FB police

New profiles generated at a pinch

Touching nerves. It was a cinch

A wee rebellious rant that tells the truth

A few lines are all it took

Impossible Dreams

Impossible to touch and impossible to taste

Deep thoughts in amongst the flux of creation

Application steady and true to a dreamful destination

Somewhere the future beckons

In seconds it could be settled

It could be stardom or the crash of moondust

Boom or bust

But creation is all about heart

Second winds or second gusts

Dedication with a pulse

It's a start

Thoughts beating fast

Heart beating last

Touch the sky only to fall

Soul screaming that's not our goal

Soul screaming enriches my soul

Impossible dreams are calling

I hear the echoes in the deep

Wake up now, chase your dreams, or forever sleep

Interstellar

Soul set on the stars above

Heart forever lost in a starlit night

A problem with a solution thereof

A drive into the dark whilst seeking the light

Lost in time, the universe for tea

A cerebral journey, a launch into space

A voyage of cosmic calamity

A heartfelt dream to chase

What path will you choose?

Travelling towards that distant sun

No time to waste, no time to snooze

Cook it, aim to be number one

Shoot for the stars when the night-time falls

Hold on, hang tight, you've got the balls

Monkey Spit

Work, work, work, toil, and trouble

Westerly winds on the double

What a puzzle

Ticking boxes

Staying sane

Sprouting wings to fly again

Fly now my monkeys

Fly

Head West along that road

Don't be yellow

Don't you goad

Wicked winged creatures

Silhouettes in the sky

Flying on mass

Desperately trying to do or die

Fly my monkeys

Fly

Mutable Truths

What is the truth?

Is it just another lie?

Hard facts corrupted

Hard facts fried . . .

Someone else's perspective before we die

A learnt education that's lost in discourse

Plus, there's imagination of course

A smattering of wondering why o why?

Plus, our attempts to do or die

A strong belief in oneself misplaced

Our truth distorted by experience

By our grace

Is our truth someone else's truth?

Our feelings denied

But emotions are true for a moment,

Free for a moment

A fleeting moment

Our emotive truth concealed by insecurities

Hidden deep inside

Transient feelings our atonement for living the lie

Fairy tales collected

The truths we rejected

We started to hunt that much is true

We eat, we feed, we fuck

There are cave paintings too

Imaginations running wild

Metaphysical meat placed before us

Laid out to chew

On our existential barbecue

Nirvana's Kiss

Keep on seeking the light of life

Release those fears before desire consumes you

Freedom transcends Samsara's strife

Illumination comes out of the blue

Let go, a wise contemplation

Breathe, let the suffering slide

Right there before reincarnation

Lose your mind during this Soma glide

Beatitude beckons, a light in the distance

Embrace the emptiness, clear your mind

Enlightenment is a product of slow persistence

Free your mind from all its craziness

Free your mind for paradise and happiness

Phoenix

I hunger for another life. I want its flaming glory

To rise. To fall. To live. To die. My destiny is calling

A revival of passions. A revival of spirit

A resurgence of mind like a sparkling sun's soul

So cool. So fine. So fast. So, let it all go

Arisen from the ashes of a moonlit silence

Death, a simple device for my acts of defiance

Reset, Reboot, Restart

Down this road we've travelled today

Walking, running, until the end of days

Our journey has only just begun

We've reached the brink

Let's carry on

Just what is around the corner?

Fate it seems has tried to warn us

Some say solidify

Let's fix this hopeless chorus

Fragmented

We've seen the gaps

In our collective consciousness

I hear compassion calling out their names

Will our global reset make us change

Our whimsical ways,

Our reflections on our halcyon days?

Will it give us hope?

The future

It can't be a joke

Let's start

Let's reboot

Let's restart the game

Let's save the day

And work our way through this

Let's carry on over the horizon

Until the winter solstice has gone

Let's see tomorrow's sun bind us to our fate

Selene

In centuries past we worshiped you

Fertility gods and mothers too

Elevated up on high

A bright blue moon in a starlight sky

Selene slowly opens her midnight soul

Our mother moon serenades and soothes our home

She is light chasing the shadows alone

She is the night personified

Half, full, quarter, eclipse

Time unfolds on solstice highways

An ever-changing chariot of the celestial heavens

A midnight kiss before sweet dreams and bliss

Selene's embrace comes in many phases

Her soft light sleeping the sleep of ages

Seven

It could be argued that I'm a slob

I'm slow and lazy, there's just a hint of sloth

I have so many imperfections

I'm perfect for the job

My heart full of pride from my endeavours

I seek enlightenment from my misadventures

Should I cast my sins aside?

Should I embrace them or let them slide

Our life lessons must be found

Virtues and sins; I am abound

Our emotions governed by experience

From our acts of quiet defiance

Our emotions given from behind our shroud

We must stand out in amongst the crowd

The darkness of wrath I have become

Only to find temperance, empathy, fortitude, and fun

A new look

A new fashion

A heart felt compassion and hope for those who struggle

I am greedy for love. That's always a muddle

I see envy evolved from my lust, from my lovelorn troubles

Somewhere stuck in a repetitive bubble

A gluttony of confusion hidden in our very souls

Rejections, exceptions, love lost, and love goals

Charity, courage, a solution to loneliness

I seek justice for my forlorn heart

I seek togetherness

Is there anyone out there who'll give me a start?

Have faith, how confusing, or is it only just a dream

All too easy, or so it seems

Without it we wouldn't believe in hope

Our imperfections make us; it's no joke

Space Chase

I seek refuge from the calamity of life

Peace and harmony my only vice

Raucous laughter

Giggles and glee

Take a look and see what you can see

Awaken mid fit

Giggle. Relax

Just sit

Giggle some more

Chat galore

Find more meaning that's for sure

Turn on the music

Open some doors

Go deep

Submerge

Ping. . . Ping. . . Ping. . .

Bleep . . . Bleep . . . Bleep

Get in the zone

What is this philosopher's stone?

An elixir of life or just fun fuelled libations

One of Mother Nature's creations

Space Suit

I need air to breath

That is a must

I'm in orbit around other stars

Moons, and dust

Exploring other suits

Other worlds

Other rocketeers

Travelling on a journey

Challenging all our fears

Making oxygen connections

Spinning in a dance

Breathing

Breathing

This could be our last chance

To deprive our soul of solitude

To enhance our lonely fortitude

We have a dizzying desire

A heart on fire

I'm asking for positive reflections

Let us chatter under scrutiny

Who are these other suits we see?

Travelling around our universe

Lost until we are found

Making oxygen connections

Say hello, let's chat, that would be sound

Sparkled

Look, see me, I am laughter

I am giggles

I am sin

Undress my devilish smiles

Catch me where I spin

In amongst the sparkling moonbeams

Just dance freely when I sing

Look up

Look down

Solstice stars reflected in the blue

I see your eyes

I see your heart

I see summer shining through

Beat, pulse, beat, pulse

More pleasure

More fever

The quickening right on cue

Stuck in Da Loop

End of the road or so it seems

A heart left wanting those distant dreams

Satisfaction was never guaranteed

More work, let's make it fun

Stand up, giggle, there is work to be done

A strange indicator, a strange obsession

Save the world until it's better

A reoccurring call to inspire this sphere into action

More love needed in this transaction

More art, more poetry, more creation

More truth of hearts

A worthy contemplation

The worthiest of starts

Sugar Coated Rainbows

Star kissed

Star struck

Dumb luck a go-go

I'd love to lick a rainbow

Just to feel the sunshine on my tongue

Warm me up and colour my mind with wholesome

My favourite foods to digest

Love, peace, harmony, and anything truly scrumptious are the best

Flavours like a glittering fizz of fun

Mouth popping

Jaw dropping

Brain bopping

Fun, Yes, Fun

I'd love to lick a rainbow

Be there at the parting of the clouds

Just to catch a colourful droplet

Of faerie dust in the sun

The Atheist Angel

Can I be honest with you?

Do you want to know a secret?

I'm reaching out; I'm kinda blue

I find myself in a deep, deep, rut

Entrenched by science and such

But divinity came knocking on my door

Fuck me sideways, I've had the angel's touch

Mind blown, insights, disbelief, you know the score

But I am an angel in an old-fashioned sense

Many, many moons ago, I wore a simple circle of light

But I don't believe in God, it's all just human experience

Angels live amongst us. Could I be right?

Is it the mind that goes flying up to the heavens above?

Rising high and floating on the wings of a dove

The Covenant

Beyond the words and phrases

There lies a pact to be fulfilled

Beyond the images and mazes

Ideas lie scattered, loosened by the thrill

Time to elevate, fly down from grace

With wings caressed by apocalypse flames

Shit! GOD smacked; mind fucked all over the place

Since fire and brimstone signed your name

Thou doeth as thou are told

From now on you are a slave

Strapped in shackles that are millennia old

A job for life, until the grave

Skull driven by the sight of the immortal sun

A covenant sanctioned, an obsession has begun

The Crunch

Upon many roads I have travelled

In one direction that's perilous and narrow

Driven by a focused obsession

Driven by a dire confession

Just driven

Hell bent and heaven sent

By an avenging angel's curse

And a vision to defy all visions

Actions sanctioned by divinity

Actions blessed by stupidity

A journey into oblivion at best

A quest

Endurance

Endeavours

Endless misadventures

I have travelled

But it appears over the horizon

A choice

It's not surprising

A crossroads comes near

Will I change the world, or will I crumble in fear?

The Defiant Worm

What adventures does it seek?

Babbling journeys

A babbling sneak

A blood curdling creature

A cerebral freak

A bloodstream voyeur

Travelling for sure

Past the guts

Up the spine

Nesting inside my mind

Playing catch me

Catch me if you can

Forceful coercions thrown out fast

Just trying to be the man

Hoping it won't last

Drunk in oblivion

A singular Van Damn

Fighting for peace

I'm not a fan

My worm has made me weak

It's palace derelict, destroyed, and bleak

My mind broken

No escape

Confrontation the only cure

Another fight that's for sure

So, follow me

Back down the spine

Through the heart

Have some guts

The stomach acid will do fine

Jump in, dissolve, euthanize

It's a must

Just do or die or I'll go nuts

Goodbye cruel worm

I am victorious

The Flutter By Effect

Aim for eternity

It's the forever place to be

Follow the infinite

Follow the dreams

Flutter like a butterfly

The effect history

A future with a destiny

A traveller through time

A point of origin for all to see

A flex

A flap

A smidgeon

A breeze

A tornado I see

Point A to point B

Point B to point C

Point C to point D

Evolution's trail of dust

Beaten wings sing a wanton wanderlust

What is a butterfly?

In a human sense

Is it the icons we see just being immense?

Favourites becoming forever friends

Free thought being a legend of fortune and providence

Icons making their mark on humanity

Singing future songs to be free

Too many to list

Too many to see

Elvis songs: He banged a gong

Madonna's sweet melodies

Buddha's adventures overseas

Flutter by for an eternity

Socratic philosophy in the mix

Don't forget Davinci's tricks

Creation running wild and on the loose

Dare I mention the golden goose?

Human divinity travels with providence

Sometimes it makes no sense

But butterflies are just so cool

Chaos theory's star struck fools

A festival of humanity

So, sing

Sing their songs

Come sing with me

Be a legend

Go make fucking history

The Golden Path

Does the cosmos conspire against you?

Do you believe in fate?

A legion of coincidences can only beckon the brave

Follow the path

Albeit golden

An adventure has been attained

Forget hardship

Forget pain

Forget oblivion

They are one and the same

Stand up, get back up again

Drive yourself to destiny

You'll never be the same

Seek wisdom from all that is wrong

Revel in this bloody crying game

Touch fire

Touch the moon

Touch the bonds of lunacy

Touch your future dreams

Smile and be misunderstood

But follow your calling

Don't chew on the cud

Chew on the good

Travel; follow the years one by one

Nothing stops until you are done

Chasing immortality

Chasing the setting sun

Is this glory just over the hill?

The Grudge

Fuck you, you fucking bastard

You're the bane of my existence

A nemesis slithers past us

Nagging away with every insistence

Corrupting my heart with subversive resistance

I fucking hate you

I want to destroy you

You are my poison

My life married to adrenaline

Double motherfucker fucker

You fucked me big time my old friend

A blundering muppet until the end

Fuck wit, nit wit, dim wit, stupid

Flung together by an endarkened cupid

An arrow in the mind

A splinter for all time

Your legacy of being unkind

Fuck you cunt

Do you hear me, are you fucking blind?

I hate you with my bitter heart

Something you instilled right from the start

Hatred compounded

Revulsions are moulded

Three years in this crucible called life

Three years of head fucking strife

Your people skills have made me ill

Careless words, I've had my fill

Boom, adrenal dynamite

Boom, adrenal oblivion

Boom, a Battle Royale with the slithering snake

Fuck you and fuck you still

It took years of persistence to change my will

But my nemesis still remains

A memory of darker days

My bitterness still endures

A scar on my psyche that only medication can cure

Fuck off you cunt

You soul violator

Get back in the sewer where you belong

I hope you're dead or it won't be long

Begone you bastard, begone

(Dedicated to Dr Dodds. My first Consultant Psychiatrist aka The Victorian Death. I never knew what hate was until I met you.)

The Look

Is it in the eyes?

These reflections of soul

Dark moods. Dark skies. Cynicisms to be told

Which can only be seen whilst seeking

The lights from our survival; our glory days of old.

Our calamities.

Our chaos

Our show biz shows.

Our inner child longing,

Laughing,

Craving merriment and joy,

A yearning for our friends,

A lover's love found from our hordes of souls.

A lover's love that's as good as gold

A yearning for the stories that are yet untold.

At what point did we become self-aware?

That we, the chaos, should not despair

Our innocence tarnished by these temporal flares

Our sight smudged by all things dared

Some deemed unjust,

Some deemed unfair

I'm looking steadfast, seeking,

Travelling headfirst into one more day

One more birthday is on its way

Let's go out to play in adulthood

Our inner child gone for good

Or so they say

The Taming Of The New

Embrace, drink, swagger, fill your very soul

With empty vessel troubles already written in stone

Warm the heart with effervescent bubbles

Get drunk, lick from the bottom of that singing bowl

Chant, I'm in love with me and I'm in love with all

Ego parading in the mirror before that sudden fall

Quick tempered explanations made in error when your ego calls

"You talking to me?"

"You talking to me?"

"You talking to me?"

Boozy reflections reworked for terror when your ego stalls

Self-serving insights that are substance found

Zap! Zap! Zap!

The snapped crackle of a lightning forks hitting the ground

The powers of Zeus penetrating that sobering skull

Just one more little dram

Just one more little thrill

Aim for the stars when the gutter is found

Raise your arm up to the sky

Push it and cry "I am invincible!"

Backed by flashing plasma pounding through your heart

Deep thought can only be admissible

But red alert, a deepening philosophy: life is art

Legless opinions challenged by reality

Ass quickly immobilised by gravity

Body spreadeagled on the ground

When the quickening pulses through your veins

Intoxicating spirits bludgeon the midnight brain

Thud!

Will this merrymaking ever be the same?

Watch me wake, I'll never drink again

Unknown Destinations

Where have we been and where are we going?

Through one more wall of hate

Not knowing

It's a little too late

To purge the system

Blood glistening

Between the cracks

Bitterness bleeds

And that's a fact

But time carries on regardless

I seek peace

I seek patience

I seek enlightenment through the ages

I seek

I seek

I seek

An unknown destination

Destiny calling nirvana is here,

Nirvana is here,

Nirvana is here

Like a Siren's tongue that's teasing

Come find me until your soul is bleeding

Freedom awaits the wayward and willing

Unknown Futures

I stand at the beginning of a new dream

At its heart the world

One worth saving it seems

A tease. A little twist of fate

The clock spring unravelled

Missions completed, I'm all up to date

A heart empty of purpose

Yesterday's dreams fulfilled

I sit here overwhelmed

By the demons I've killed

But there are new dreams of late

Dig deep, there's no escape

A simple glimpse of madness awaiting fate

Bygone days behind me

An apprenticeship for finding fate

20 years of wandering with experience

Acquiring skills to create,

But still way out of shape

I may be too late

Looking upwards at the legend I should be

One small step is all I need to take

Ascend the mountains once again

And cross the desert to satisfaction's gate

Waiting For Changes

We're all waiting for the change

Slow and steady work can't be blamed

Effort, resolve, be steadfast, we will win again

Wisdom from our turmoil's

Wisdom buried deep down in our hearts

Found frolicking like a lark

Waiting in a cage

To be released on the day of days

This is only the start

Slow steady work can't be blamed

We can beat this virus at its own game

But will our world ever be the same?

I hope for art, love, music, and flame

To show itself once more again

Walking With Friends

I miss him you know. My friend the talker

Yip, yap, zingy chat, and all that crap

I used to listen endlessly

He was relentless verbally

We were well suited as friends

He used to drive me round the bend

Conspiracy theories that would never end

Mother Nature a top priority

Kill all humans

His wandering war cry

He had a point

Doobies sparked in nature's awe

We used to stop, rest, and talk some more

Sometimes I could only manage an "Aye"

Just enough to keep us going

Just enough to keep the sun in the sky

One step forward to keep us on track

Through the woods

Along to the lagoon

Down the foreshore with a loon

We were well matched mentally

We used to bath in nature's serenity

Inspired by her spiritual presence

Silence in awe of tranquillity

Walking by lake or reservoir

Saying hello to those that were friendly

I miss wee Stuart. I miss him endlessly

Weekly Chores

Trying to write a poem a week

Easy said but this is no mean feat

My muse is starving, slippery, and sleek

She's just out there

Just out of reach

Love without hate

Smiles, emotions, fate

Colours and hues

Songs sung sweet with cathartic blues

Friendships found

Friendships lost

A bared soul is the creative cost

Of poetry

A rippling heart is an existential fuss

Put those words down

So they can be found

It's a must

Infuse a heart with passion

Infuse a heart with sorrow

Infuse a heart tomorrow

Come together

Poets unite

Before we all turn to dust

We Should Be Dancing

Bands blaring out a salacious beat

Hips ready; wiggle it, swing that ass

Pound that meat

Let the music lose you

In a pulse

In a dream

In a heartbeat

Sounds travelling right down through your soul

Right down to your feet

Deep drums pounding

A hi hat cracking

Beat, beat, beat

Absolute abandon amassing

Pleasing

Teasing

Let the music move you

Caress you

Run your hands upwards along your thighs

Raise them up into the electric sky

It's such a sexy beat

Head whipped back

Flung side to side

There it is. There's that smile

Let's all go to one more gig

It's been a while

What is Love?

Love could be what we cannot see

Butterflies inside the gut tickling and such

A blush from a smile from an invisible glee

A heart flowing with that fantasia touch

Love is pure. Love is love. Love is fire in the blood

Love is gazing at a perfect angel's face

Love is gazing at a handsome stud

Love is chemistry all over the place

Drunk love. A little sip. Just enough to make you blind

Lost in a passion that's always divine

Love is the only thing in this world to find

Follow your instinct to embrace the sublime

Need I mention the moon on a starlit night?

Stunning, I have to say you're just out of sight

Whimsical

After every intension has been burned

I find myself in a space

I need to breathe

I need to reflect on what has been done

Has anything changed?

Has the slip knot been pulled?

Have people been schooled enough to understand?

Education, a form of letting go

If I'd only known the things I know now

But flippant moods suggest progress

I should smile more and worry less

There is a bridge to happiness

I call it melancholic fun

Something that just has to be done

A quiet victory in your mind

Smile and try to be kind

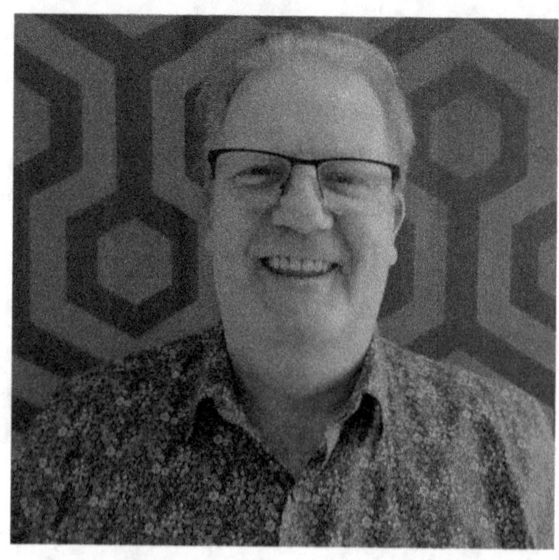

Hi folks, I've been writing for several years now. Mainly as a hobby writer but I do have the writer's dream of writing a popular book. Over the years I've been published in a few places: Quailbell Magazine, The Scottish Book Trust, The Falkirk Herald newspaper, Asylum Magazine, and some of my art has been published in an online magazine called: Paper Dragon, a Drexel University publication, (Philadelphia). I should also include the various For the Many Not the Few publications that I've been part of. Especially my first book: Red Pill Memories. Plus, I have to include my Express Yourself on the radio antics. Express Yourself being the title of a Sunny Govan radio show for poets. I've sent in a few poems in to be aired and I sound terrible. I've also performed at various spoken word events within the Falkirk area. My attitude to creativity is the slow and steady approach mixed with outbursts of inspiration. I like to keep it fun with my poetry and writing. If I make someone smile, I'm happy too. Did I mention my abstract art? I've been plodding along with that for years too.

Steven
July
2022

---

*My acknowledgements go to Meek at Inherit The Earth (Online Publications)
and to my Community Psychiatric Nurse, Yvonne.*

Steven Joseph McCrystal

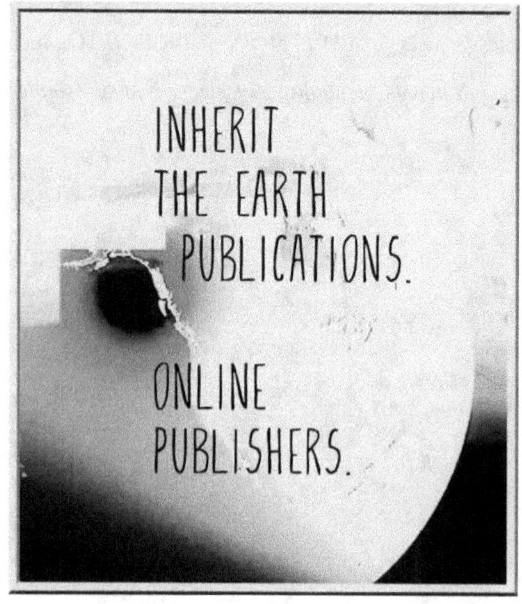

inherit_theearth@btbtinternet.com

Notes